STARVE CANCER WITH FOOD

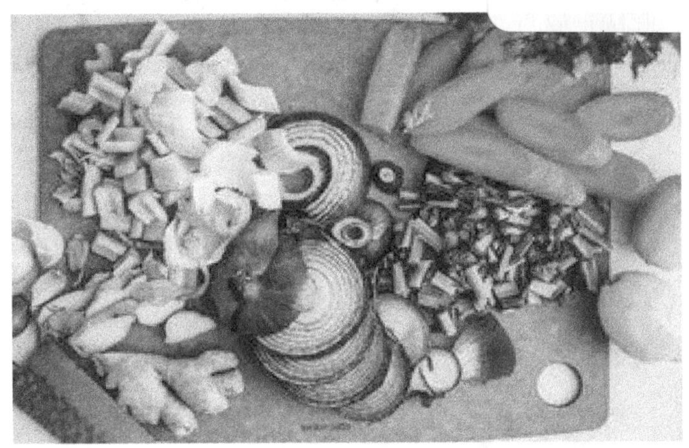

Nutritious and Healthy Whole-Food
Cancer-Fighting Recipes for Managing
Recovery and Reducing Cancer Risk
(Including Meal Plan and Tips)

By

Dr. Clara Ramsey

Table of Contents

5 | STARVE CANCER WITH FOOD

Introduction

Cancer remains one of the most formidable health challenges of our time, affecting millions of lives worldwide. While advancements in medical science have led to improved treatment options and survival rates, the quest for effective prevention strategies remains paramount. In this pursuit, the role of diet has emerged as a powerful ally in the fight against cancer.

The concept of starving cancer with food revolves around the idea that certain foods and dietary patterns may influence the development and progression of cancer.

Research suggests that consuming a variety of nutrient-rich foods, while minimizing intake of processed and unhealthy options, can help lower cancer risk and improve overall health outcomes.

The foundation to starve cancer with food lies in promoting whole, plant-based foods abundant in vitamins, minerals, antioxidants, and phytonutrients.

These natural compounds have been shown to possess anti-inflammatory, antioxidant, and anti-carcinogenic properties, which can help protect cells from damage and reduce the risk of cancer formation.

At the heart of the starve cancer with food is the emphasis on a diverse array of fruits, vegetables, whole grains, legumes, nuts, seeds, and lean protein sources. These foods provide essential nutrients and bioactive compounds that support immune function, regulate inflammation, and promote cellular repair and regeneration.

Conversely, the starve cancer with food advises against the consumption of processed foods, sugary snacks, red and processed meats, refined grains, and high-fat dairy products.

These items have been linked to increased inflammation, oxidative stress, and disruptions in metabolic health, which may contribute to cancer development and progression.

While diet alone cannot guarantee immunity from cancer, adopting a balanced and nutritious eating pattern is proactive step individuals can take to reduce their risk.

Moreover, for those already diagnosed with cancer, a supportive anti-cancer diet can complement medical treatments, enhance quality of life, and improve treatment outcomes.

9 | STARVE CANCER WITH FOOD

In this comprehensive guide, we delve into the principles of the anti-cancer diet, explore the science behind its effectiveness, and provide practical tips and resources to help you incorporate cancer-fighting foods into your daily life. Whether you're seeking to prevent cancer, support your journey to recovery, or simply embrace a healthier lifestyle, starving cancer with food offers a roadmap to empowerment and well-being. Together, let us embark on this journey towards optimal health and resilience against cancer.

Chapter One

Cancer and Nutrition

Cancer is a complex disease characterized by the uncontrolled growth and spread of abnormal cells within the body. It can arise in virtually any organ or tissue and is influenced by a multitude of genetic, environmental, and lifestyle factors.

While genetics play a significant role in determining cancer risk, emerging research suggests that modifiable lifestyle factors, including diet, may also play a crucial role in cancer development, progression, and management.

Nutrition is intricately linked to cancer biology, with dietary choices exerting profound effects on cellular metabolism, inflammation, immune function, and gene expression. While no single food or nutrient can prevent or cure cancer, evidence suggests that certain dietary patterns and components may influence cancer risk and prognosis.

Key factors linking nutrition and cancer include:

Inflammation: Chronic inflammation is a hallmark of cancer development and progression. Certain dietary patterns, such as those high in processed foods, refined sugars, and unhealthy fats, can promote systemic inflammation, creating an environment conducive to cancer growth.

Conversely, anti-inflammatory foods, such as fruits, vegetables, whole grains, and omega-3 fatty acids, may help mitigate inflammation and reduce cancer risk.

Oxidative Stress: Reactive oxygen species (ROS), produced during cellular metabolism, can cause oxidative damage to DNA, proteins, and lipids, contributing to cancer initiation and progression. Antioxidants, found abundantly in colorful fruits, vegetables, and plant-based foods, help neutralize ROS and protect cells from oxidative damage, potentially lowering cancer risk.

Immune Function: The immune system plays a critical role in cancer surveillance and defense, identifying and eliminating abnormal cells before they can proliferate and form tumors.

Nutrient-rich foods, such as vitamin C, vitamin E, zinc, and selenium, support immune function and enhance the body's ability to combat cancer cells.

Hormonal Balance: Certain cancers, such as breast and prostate cancer, are influenced by hormonal factors. Dietary components, such as phytoestrogens found in soybeans and flaxseeds, may modulate hormone levels and reduce cancer risk in hormonally sensitive tissues.

Microbiome: The gut microbiome, comprised of trillions of bacteria and other microorganisms, plays a crucial role in immune function, inflammation, and metabolism.

Emerging research suggests that dietary factors can influence the composition and diversity of the microbiome, which, in turn, may impact cancer risk and progression.

By understanding the intricate interplay between nutrition and cancer biology, individuals can make informed dietary choices to reduce their risk of cancer and support overall health.

A balanced diet rich in fruits, vegetables, whole grains, lean proteins, and healthy fats serves as the foundation of a cancer-preventive lifestyle. Moreover, adopting healthy eating habits, such as maintaining a healthy weight, limiting alcohol consumption, and avoiding tobacco use, can further enhance cancer prevention efforts.

In the following sections, we will explore specific dietary components, patterns, and strategies that have been associated with cancer prevention and management. Through education, empowerment, and proactive lifestyle modifications, we can harness the power of nutrition to promote health, resilience, and vitality in the face of cancer.

The Role of Diet in Cancer Prevention and Treatment

Diet plays a crucial role in cancer prevention and treatment, influencing various biological processes that contribute to cancer development, progression, and response to therapy.

While genetics and environmental factors also play significant roles in cancer risk, emerging research highlights the powerful impact of dietary choices on cancer outcomes.

Understanding the role of diet in cancer prevention and treatment can empower individuals to make informed choices that support overall health and well-being.

Cancer Prevention

Epidemiological studies have consistently shown associations between certain dietary patterns and cancer risk. A diet rich in fruits, vegetables, whole grains, and lean proteins is associated with a lower risk of several types of cancer, including colorectal, breast, prostate, and lung cancer.

Plant-based foods are abundant in phytonutrients, antioxidants, vitamins, and minerals that possess anti-inflammatory, antioxidant, and anti-carcinogenic properties. These compounds help neutralize free radicals, reduce inflammation, and protect cells from DNA damage, thereby lowering cancer risk.

Conversely, diets high in processed foods, red and processed meats, sugary beverages, and unhealthy fats have been linked to an increased risk of cancer. These foods may promote inflammation, oxidative stress, insulin resistance, and dysbiosis, creating an environment conducive to cancer growth and progression.

Cancer Treatment Support

Nutrition plays a critical role in supporting cancer treatment outcomes and enhancing quality of life for individuals undergoing therapy. Adequate nutrition helps maintain immune function, preserve lean body mass, reduce treatment-related side effects, and improve overall tolerance to therapy.

Cancer treatments such as chemotherapy, radiation therapy, and surgery can impact appetite, taste perception, digestion, and nutrient absorption. Nutritional interventions, including dietary modifications, nutritional supplementation, and supportive care, can help address these challenges and optimize nutritional status during treatment.

Certain dietary components, such as omega-3 fatty acids, glutamine, arginine, and antioxidants, may have potential benefits in mitigating treatment-related toxicities, reducing inflammation, and supporting tissue repair and recovery.

However, individualized dietary recommendations should be tailored to the specific needs and tolerances of each patient, taking into account their cancer type, treatment regimen, and nutritional status.

Survivorship and Long-Term Health

Beyond the acute phase of treatment, nutrition continues to play a vital role in cancer survivorship and long-term health.

Adopting a balanced and nutrient-rich diet can help mitigate the risk of cancer recurrence, promote overall wellness, and reduce the risk of comorbid conditions such as cardiovascular disease, diabetes, and obesity.

Lifestyle factors, including diet, physical activity, weight management, and tobacco cessation, are key determinants of long-term health outcomes among cancer survivors. Integrating healthy habits into daily life can support optimal recovery, resilience, and quality of life after cancer treatment.

In general diet plays a multifaceted role in cancer prevention, treatment, and survivorship. By prioritizing a plant-based diet rich in fruits, vegetables, whole grains, and lean proteins, individuals can harness the power of nutrition to reduce cancer risk, support treatment efficacy, and promote long-term health and well-being.

Moreover, ongoing research and collaboration among healthcare professionals, researchers, and patients are essential to further elucidate the complex interactions between diet, cancer biology, and therapeutic outcomes.

Through education, advocacy, and proactive lifestyle modifications, we can empower individuals to take charge of their health and make informed choices that contribute to cancer prevention and treatment success.

Chapter Two

Benefits of Starving Cancer with Food

Reduced Cancer Risk:

One of the primary benefits of adopting an anti-cancer diet is a reduction in cancer risk. Research suggests that certain dietary patterns and components can influence the development and progression of cancer.

By emphasizing whole, nutrient-rich foods and minimizing intake of processed and unhealthy options, individuals can lower their risk of developing various types of cancer, including colorectal, breast, prostate, lung, and stomach cancer.

Antioxidant Protection:

An anti-cancer diet is rich in antioxidants, which are compounds that help neutralize harmful free radicals and oxidative stress in the body. Free radicals are unstable molecules that can damage cells and DNA, leading to inflammation, oxidative damage, and increased cancer risk.

Antioxidant-rich foods such as fruits, vegetables, nuts, seeds, and legumes help protect cells from oxidative damage and support overall health and well-being.

Anti-Inflammatory Effects:

Chronic inflammation is a key driver of cancer development and progression. An anti-cancer diet emphasizes foods that have anti-inflammatory properties, such as fruits, vegetables, whole grains, and omega-3 fatty acids.

These foods help reduce inflammation in the body, creating an environment that is less conducive to cancer growth and metastasis.

Immune Support:

The immune system plays a critical role in cancer surveillance and defense, identifying and eliminating abnormal cells before they can proliferate and form tumors. Certain nutrients, such as vitamin C, vitamin E, zinc, selenium, and phytonutrients, support immune function and enhance the body's ability to combat cancer cells.

By consuming a diet rich in immune-boosting nutrients, individuals can strengthen their immune system and improve their ability to prevent and fight cancer.

Regulation of Hormonal Balance:

Hormonal imbalances can contribute to the development and progression of certain types of cancer, such as breast and prostate cancer. An anti-cancer diet includes foods that help regulate hormonal balance, such as phytoestrogens found in soybeans, flaxseeds, and legumes.

These plant-based compounds can modulate hormone levels and reduce the risk of hormonally driven cancers.

Maintenance of Healthy Weight:

Obesity and excess body fat have been linked to an increased risk of several types of cancer, including breast, colorectal, endometrial, and kidney cancer. An anti-cancer diet emphasizes nutrient-dense, low-calorie foods that promote satiety, regulate appetite, and support weight management.

By adopting healthy eating habits and maintaining a healthy weight, individuals can reduce their risk of obesity-related cancers and improve overall health outcomes.

Improved Overall Health:

In addition to reducing cancer risk, an anti-cancer diet offers numerous benefits for overall health and well-being. By prioritizing whole, minimally processed foods and avoiding harmful dietary components, individuals can improve their cardiovascular health, blood sugar control, digestive function, and mental well-being.

A balanced and nutritious diet supports optimal health outcomes and enhances resilience against chronic diseases, including cancer.

For short, the benefits of an anti-cancer diet extend far beyond cancer prevention. By nourishing the body with nutrient-rich foods, supporting immune function, and reducing inflammation and oxidative stress, individuals can optimize their health and well-being while lowering their risk of cancer and other chronic diseases.

Embracing a plant-based diet rich in fruits, vegetables, whole grains, and lean proteins serves as a powerful tool for promoting longevity, vitality, and resilience against cancer and other health challenges.

Understanding Cancer and Its Risk Factors

As I said earlier, cancer is a complex and multifaceted group of diseases characterized by the uncontrolled growth and spread of abnormal cells within the body. Normal cells in the body grow, divide, and die in a regulated manner as part of the body's natural processes of growth, repair, and maintenance.

However, in cancer, this orderly process is disrupted, leading to the formation of malignant tumors or abnormal cell masses.

Key Features of Cancer:

Uncontrolled Cell Growth: Cancer begins when genetic mutations or alterations occur within the DNA of a cell, disrupting its normal function and causing it to divide and proliferate uncontrollably.

These mutations can be caused by various factors, including environmental exposures, lifestyle habits, genetic predispositions, and random errors in cell division.

Formation of Tumors: As cancer cells continue to multiply, they can form tumors or abnormal growths within tissues or organs.

Tumors may be localized or invasive, and they can interfere with normal bodily functions depending on their size, location, and characteristics.

Invasion and Metastasis: In addition to local growth, cancer cells have the ability to invade nearby tissues and organs, infiltrate blood vessels or lymphatic channels, and spread to distant parts of the body.

This process, known as metastasis, is a hallmark of cancer progression and is responsible for the majority of cancer-related deaths.

Heterogeneity and Adaptation: Cancer is characterized by heterogeneity, meaning that tumors are composed of a diverse population of cancer cells with varying genetic, molecular, and phenotypic characteristics.

This heterogeneity enables cancer cells to adapt to changing environments, evade immune detection, resist treatment, and survive under adverse conditions.

Interaction with the Microenvironment: Cancer cells interact with their surrounding microenvironment, which includes blood vessels, immune cells, fibroblasts, and extracellular matrix components.

These interactions play a crucial role in cancer progression, metastasis, and response to therapy.

Common Types of Cancer

Cancer is a diverse group of diseases, with more than 100 different types identified based on the tissues or organs in which they originate. Each type of cancer has unique characteristics, behaviors, risk factors, and treatment approaches.

Understanding the most common types of cancer is essential for raising awareness, promoting early detection, and improving outcomes for affected individuals. Here are some of the most prevalent types of cancer:

Breast Cancer:

Breast cancer occurs when abnormal cells develop in the breast tissue. It is the most common cancer among women worldwide and can also affect men.

Risk factors for breast cancer include family history, genetic mutations (such as BRCA1 and BRCA2), age, hormonal factors, obesity, alcohol consumption, and exposure to radiation.

Early detection through regular mammograms and clinical breast exams, along with self-examination, is crucial for improving survival rates.

Lung Cancer:

Lung cancer begins in the cells of the lungs and is primarily caused by tobacco smoking, although non-smokers can also develop the disease due to exposure to secondhand smoke, air pollution, radon gas, and occupational carcinogens.

There are two main types of lung cancer: non-small cell lung cancer (NSCLC) and small cell lung cancer (SCLC), each with different characteristics and treatment options.

Symptoms of lung cancer may include persistent cough, chest pain, shortness of breath, coughing up blood, fatigue, and unexplained weight loss.

Colorectal Cancer:

Colorectal cancer affects the colon or rectum and usually develops from precancerous polyps in the lining of the colon or rectum.

Risk factors for colorectal cancer include age, family history, personal history of inflammatory bowel disease or colorectal polyps, diet high in red and processed meats, low fiber intake, sedentary lifestyle, obesity, smoking, and heavy alcohol consumption.

Screening tests such as colonoscopies, fecal occult blood tests, and stool DNA tests can help detect colorectal cancer early when it is most treatable.

Prostate Cancer:

Prostate cancer develops in the prostate gland, which is located below the bladder and in front of the rectum in men. It is the most common cancer among men, particularly older men.

Risk factors for prostate cancer include age, family history, African American ethnicity, and certain genetic mutations.

Screening for prostate cancer involves a prostate-specific antigen (PSA) blood test and digital rectal examination, although the benefits and risks of screening are still debated.

Skin Cancer (Melanoma and Non-Melanoma):

Skin cancer is the abnormal growth of skin cells, and it is primarily caused by exposure to ultraviolet (UV) radiation from the sun or tanning beds.

Melanoma is the most dangerous form of skin cancer and can spread quickly if not detected early. Non-melanoma skin cancers, such as basal cell carcinoma and squamous cell carcinoma, are more common but less likely to spread.

Prevention strategies for skin cancer include wearing sunscreen, protective clothing, and sunglasses, seeking shade, and avoiding indoor tanning.

Leukemia:

Leukemia is a cancer of the blood and bone marrow, characterized by the overproduction of abnormal white blood cells. It affects both children and adults.

There are several types of leukemia, including acute lymphoblastic leukemia (ALL), acute myeloid leukemia (AML), chronic lymphocytic leukemia (CLL), and chronic myeloid leukemia (CML), each with different features and treatment approaches.

Symptoms of leukemia may include fatigue, weakness, frequent infections, easy bruising or bleeding, swollen lymph nodes, and unexplained weight loss.

These are just a few examples of the most common types of cancer, but many other types exist, each with its own unique characteristics and challenges. Early detection, timely treatment, and ongoing research are crucial for improving outcomes and reducing the burden of cancer worldwide.

Risk Factors for Developing Cancer

Cancer is a complex disease influenced by a combination of genetic, environmental, lifestyle, and hormonal factors. While some risk factors for cancer cannot be modified, such as age and family history, many others are modifiable through lifestyle changes and preventive measures.

Understanding these risk factors is essential for raising awareness, promoting early detection, and implementing preventive strategies to reduce the incidence of cancer.

Here are some of the key risk factors associated with developing cancer:

Genetic Predisposition:

Genetic factors play a significant role in determining an individual's risk of developing cancer. Inherited genetic mutations, such as those associated with BRCA1 and BRCA2 genes in breast and ovarian cancer, Lynch syndrome in colorectal cancer, and familial adenomatous polyposis (FAP) in colon cancer, can significantly increase the likelihood of developing certain types of cancer.

Environmental Exposures:

Exposure to carcinogenic substances in the environment can increase the risk of cancer. These substances may include tobacco smoke, asbestos fibers, benzene, radon gas, arsenic, formaldehyde, and certain industrial chemicals. Occupational exposure to carcinogens in workplaces such as construction, mining, manufacturing, and agriculture can also elevate cancer risk.

Lifestyle Factors:

Unhealthy lifestyle behaviors can contribute to cancer development. These include:

- ***Tobacco Use:*** Smoking and exposure to secondhand smoke are leading causes of lung, mouth, throat, and bladder cancer. Smokeless tobacco products, such as chewing tobacco and snuff, also increase cancer risk.
- ***Poor Diet:*** A diet high in processed foods, red and processed meats, saturated fats, sugars, and low in fruits, vegetables, and fiber is associated with an increased risk of cancer, particularly colorectal, breast, and prostate cancer.

- **Physical Inactivity:** Lack of regular physical activity is linked to an increased risk of several types of cancer, including colon, breast, and endometrial cancer.

- ***Excessive Alcohol Consumption:*** Heavy alcohol consumption is associated with an elevated risk of several cancers, including liver, breast, colorectal, and esophageal cancer.

Body Weight and Obesity:

Obesity and excess body weight are significant risk factors for several types of cancer, including breast, colorectal, endometrial, kidney, pancreatic, and esophageal cancer.

Obesity is associated with chronic inflammation, insulin resistance, hormonal imbalances, and alterations in adipokine levels, all of which contribute to cancer development and progression.

Chronic Inflammation:

Chronic inflammation due to infections, autoimmune disorders, inflammatory bowel disease, or chronic exposure to environmental toxins can promote cancer development.

Inflammatory cytokines, chemokines, and reactive oxygen species produced during chronic inflammation can induce DNA damage, cellular proliferation, and genetic mutations, fostering a pro-cancerous environment.

Hormonal Factors:

Hormonal imbalances or exposures can influence cancer risk. For example, hormonal contraceptives, hormone replacement therapy, and exposure to estrogen and progesterone are associated with an increased risk of breast and ovarian cancer. Similarly, hormonal factors play a role in the development of prostate and endometrial cancer.

Infectious Agents:

Certain infectious agents, including viruses, bacteria, and parasites, are linked to an increased risk of cancer. Examples include:

Human papillomavirus (HPV): Linked to cervical, anal, penile, and oropharyngeal cancers.

Hepatitis B and C viruses: Associated with liver cancer.

Helicobacter pylori: Linked to stomach cancer.

Epstein-Barr virus (EBV): Associated with lymphoma and nasopharyngeal cancer.

By understanding these risk factors, individuals can take proactive steps to modify lifestyle behaviors, minimize exposure to environmental toxins, and undergo appropriate screening and surveillance to reduce their risk of developing cancer.

Additionally, ongoing research into the underlying mechanisms of cancer development and progression holds promise for the development of targeted prevention and treatment strategies aimed at reducing the global burden of cancer.

Chapter Three

Lifestyle Factors and Cancer Risk

Tobacco Use:

Tobacco use, including smoking cigarettes, cigars, pipes, and using smokeless tobacco products, is one of the leading causes of cancer worldwide.

Tobacco smoke contains thousands of chemicals, many of which are carcinogenic and can damage DNA, leading to the development of cancer.

Quitting smoking and avoiding exposure to secondhand smoke can significantly reduce the risk of developing various types of cancer, including lung, mouth, throat, esophagus, bladder, kidney, pancreas, and cervix cancer.

Diet and Nutrition:

41 | STARVE CANCER WITH FOOD

A poor diet high in processed foods, red and processed meats, sugary beverages, and unhealthy fats is associated with an increased risk of cancer. Conversely, a healthy diet rich in fruits, vegetables, whole grains, lean proteins, and healthy fats can lower cancer risk.

Key dietary principles for reducing cancer risk include consuming a variety of colorful fruits and vegetables, choosing whole grains over refined grains, limiting red and processed meats, avoiding sugary and processed foods, and staying hydrated by drinking plenty of water.

Physical Activity:

Regular physical activity is associated with a reduced risk of developing various types of cancer, including colon, breast, and endometrial cancer. Exercise helps maintain a healthy weight, reduces inflammation, boosts immune function, and improves hormonal balance, all of which contribute to lower cancer risk.

Aim for at least 150 minutes of moderate-intensity aerobic activity or 75 minutes of vigorous-intensity activity per week, along with muscle-strengthening exercises on two or more days per week.

Body Weight and Obesity:

Obesity and excess body weight are significant risk factors for several types of cancer, including breast, colorectal, endometrial, kidney, pancreatic, and esophageal cancer.

Obesity is associated with chronic inflammation, insulin resistance, hormonal imbalances, and altered metabolism, all of which promote cancer development and progression.

Achieving and maintaining a healthy weight through a balanced diet and regular physical activity can help reduce cancer risk and improve overall health outcomes.

Alcohol Consumption:

Heavy alcohol consumption is linked to an increased risk of several types of cancer, including liver, breast, colorectal, esophageal, and oral cancer. Alcohol can damage DNA, disrupt hormone levels, impair immune function, and promote inflammation, all of which contribute to cancer development.

Limit alcohol consumption to moderate levels: up to one drink per day for women and up to two drinks per day for men.

Key Principles of the Anti-Cancer Diet

Emphasize Plant-Based Foods:

Fruits, vegetables, whole grains, legumes, nuts, and seeds are rich in vitamins, minerals, antioxidants, and phytochemicals that help protect against cancer. Aim to fill half your plate with colorful plant foods at each meal.

Choose Healthy Fats:

Opt for healthy fats from sources such as olive oil, avocado, nuts, and seeds, while limiting saturated and trans fats found in red and processed meats, fried foods, and processed snacks.

Limit Red and Processed Meats:

Red and processed meats, such as beef, pork, lamb, bacon, sausage, and deli meats, are associated with an increased risk of cancer, particularly colorectal cancer. Limit intake and choose lean protein sources such as poultry, fish, beans, and lentils.

Minimize Sugary and Processed Foods:

Sugary beverages, sweets, processed snacks, and refined carbohydrates can contribute to weight gain, inflammation, and insulin resistance, increasing cancer risk. Choose whole, unprocessed foods whenever possible and limit added sugars in your diet.

Stay Hydrated:

Drink plenty of water throughout the day to stay hydrated and support overall health and well-being. Limit consumption of sugary beverages and opt for water, herbal tea, or sparkling water instead.

By incorporating these lifestyle factors and dietary principles into your daily routine, you can help reduce your risk of developing cancer and improve your overall health and well-being. Remember that small changes can add up over time, so focus on making sustainable lifestyle modifications that you can maintain for the long term.

Overview of the Anti-Cancer Diet

The anti-cancer diet is a dietary approach focused on promoting health and reducing the risk of cancer by emphasizing whole, nutrient-rich foods while avoiding harmful substances.

This dietary pattern prioritizes plant-based foods, lean proteins, healthy fats, and a variety of fruits, vegetables, whole grains, nuts, seeds, and legumes.

By adopting an anti-cancer diet, individuals can optimize their nutritional intake, support immune function, reduce inflammation, and create an internal environment that is less conducive to cancer development and progression.

Emphasizing Whole Foods:

Whole foods are minimally processed and retain their natural nutrients, fiber, and phytochemicals, making them essential components of the anti-cancer diet.

Emphasizing whole foods allows individuals to maximize their intake of vitamins, minerals, antioxidants, and other bioactive compounds that possess anti-inflammatory, antioxidant, and anti-carcinogenic properties. Examples of whole foods include:

- **Fruits:** Berries, citrus fruits, apples, pears, kiwi, mango, etc.
- **Vegetables:** Leafy greens, cruciferous vegetables (broccoli, kale, Brussels sprouts), carrots, bell peppers, tomatoes, etc.
- **Whole grains:** Quinoa, brown rice, barley, oats, whole wheat, millet, etc.
- **Legumes:** Beans, lentils, chickpeas, peas, etc.
- **Nuts and seeds:** Almonds, walnuts, chia seeds, flaxseeds, pumpkin seeds, etc.

Incorporating Cancer-Fighting Nutrients:

Certain nutrients found in plant-based foods have been shown to have cancer-fighting properties and may help reduce the risk of cancer. These include:

- **Antioxidants:** Found in brightly colored fruits and vegetables, antioxidants help neutralize harmful free radicals and protect cells from oxidative damage.

- **Phytochemicals:** Plant compounds such as polyphenols, flavonoids, and carotenoids have anti-inflammatory and anti-carcinogenic effects. Examples include resveratrol in grapes and berries, curcumin in turmeric, and lycopene in tomatoes.

- **Fiber:** Found in whole grains, fruits, vegetables, and legumes, dietary fiber promotes digestive health, regulates blood sugar levels, and may reduce the risk of colorectal cancer.

- ***Omega-3 fatty acids:*** Found in fatty fish (salmon, mackerel, sardines), flaxseeds, chia seeds, and walnuts, omega-3 fatty acids have anti-inflammatory properties and may help reduce the risk of certain cancers.

Avoiding Harmful Substances:

In addition to emphasizing whole foods and cancer-fighting nutrients, the anti-cancer diet emphasizes avoiding harmful substances that can increase cancer risk. These include:

- ***Processed and red meats:*** Consumption of processed meats (such as bacon, sausage, and deli meats) and red meats (such as beef, pork, and lamb) is associated with an increased risk of colorectal cancer.
- ***Sugary beverages and added sugars:*** High intake of sugary beverages, sweets, and processed

snacks has been linked to an increased risk of obesity, type 2 diabetes, and certain cancers, including breast and colorectal cancer.

- ***Trans fats and unhealthy oils:*** Trans fats found in fried foods, baked goods, and processed snacks have been linked to inflammation, heart disease, and cancer. Instead, opt for healthy fats such as olive oil, avocado oil, and nuts.

- ***Excessive alcohol consumption:*** Heavy alcohol consumption is associated with an increased risk of several types of cancer, including breast, liver, colorectal, and esophageal cancer. Limit alcohol intake to reduce cancer risk.

By incorporating these principles into their dietary habits, individuals can adopt an anti-cancer diet that supports overall health, reduces cancer risk, and promotes longevity and well-being. Additionally, combining a healthy diet with regular physical activity, maintaining a healthy weight, avoiding tobacco, and undergoing appropriate cancer screening can further enhance cancer prevention efforts.

Foods to Include in the Anti-Cancer Diet

Fruits and Vegetables: Colorful fruits and vegetables are rich in vitamins, minerals, antioxidants, and fiber, making them essential components of the anti-cancer diet.

Aim to include a variety of fruits and vegetables in your diet, focusing on dark leafy greens, berries, citrus fruits, cruciferous vegetables (such as broccoli, cauliflower, and Brussels sprouts), and colorful peppers.

Whole Grains: Whole grains provide fiber, vitamins, minerals, and phytonutrients that can help reduce cancer risk. Choose whole grains such as brown rice, quinoa, oats, barley, whole wheat, and bulgur over refined grains.

Lean Proteins: Choose lean as protein sources such as poultry, fish, tofu, tempeh, legumes, and lentils. These protein sources are rich in nutrients and lower in saturated fat than red and processed meats.

Healthy Fats: Include healthy fats in your diet from sources such as olive oil, avocado, nuts, seeds, and fatty fish. These fats provide essential fatty acids, vitamins, and antioxidants that support overall health and may help reduce inflammation.

Herbs and Spices: Herbs and spices not only add flavor to your meals but also provide potent antioxidants and anti-inflammatory compounds. Incorporate herbs and spices such as turmeric, ginger, garlic, cinnamon, and oregano into your cooking whenever possible.

Foods to Avoid in the Anti-Cancer Diet

Processed and Red Meats: Limit consumption of processed meats such as bacon, sausage, hot dogs, and deli meats, as well as red meats such as beef, pork, and lamb. These meats are high in saturated fat, cholesterol, and preservatives, and their consumption has been linked to an increased risk of colorectal cancer.

Sugary Beverages and Added Sugars: Reduce intake of sugary beverages such as soda, fruit juices, energy drinks, and sweetened teas, as well as foods high in added sugars such as candies, pastries, and desserts. High sugar intake is associated with obesity, inflammation, and an increased risk of certain cancers.

Trans Fats and Unhealthy Oils: Avoid foods made with partially hydrogenated oils, as they contain harmful trans fats that increase inflammation and promote cancer development. Limit consumption of fried foods, baked goods, and processed snacks made with unhealthy oils.

Alcohol: Limit alcohol consumption, as heavy drinking is associated with an increased risk of several types of cancer, including breast, liver, colorectal, and esophageal cancer. If you choose to drink alcohol, do so in moderation, with no more than one drink per day for women and two drinks per day for men.

Highly Processed and Ultra-Processed Foods: Minimize consumption of highly processed and ultra-processed foods such as fast food, frozen meals, chips, crackers, and packaged snacks, as these foods are often high in unhealthy fats, sugars, salt, and additives that can increase cancer risk.

By following these guidelines and incorporating a variety of nutrient-rich foods into your diet while avoiding harmful substances, you can support your body's natural defenses against cancer and promote overall health and well-being.

Remember to focus on overall dietary patterns rather than individual foods or nutrients, and strive for balance, variety, and moderation in your eating habits.

Chapter Four

Breakfast Recipes

Here are some breakfast recipes tailored to the Starve cancer with food, featuring nutrient-rich ingredients and cancer-fighting properties:

Berry and Spinach Smoothie

Ingredients:

1 cup fresh spinach leaves

1/2 cup mixed berries (such as strawberries, blueberries, and raspberries)

1/2 banana

1/2 cup Greek yogurt

1 tablespoon chia seeds

1/2 cup unsweetened almond milk

Instructions:

Combine all ingredients in a blender.

Blend until smooth and creamy.

Pour into a glass and enjoy immediately.

Avocado Toast with Poached Egg

Ingredients:

1 slice whole grain bread, toasted

1/2 ripe avocado, mashed

1 poached egg

Salt and pepper to taste

Optional toppings: sliced tomato, micro greens, red pepper flakes

Instructions:

Spread mashed avocado evenly on the toasted bread.

Top with a poached egg.

Season with salt and pepper, and add optional toppings if desired.

Serve immediately.

Quinoa Breakfast Bowl

Ingredients:

1/2 cup cooked quinoa

1/4 cup plain Greek yogurt

1/2 cup mixed berries (such as strawberries, blueberries, and raspberries)

1 tablespoon honey or maple syrup

1 tablespoon chopped nuts or seeds (such as almonds, walnuts, or chia seeds)

Instructions:

In a bowl, layer cooked quinoa, Greek yogurt, and mixed berries.

Drizzle with honey or maple syrup.

Sprinkle with chopped nuts or seeds.

Serve chilled or at room temperature.

Turmeric Oatmeal with Almonds and Honey

Ingredients:

1/2 cup rolled oats

1 cup water or milk of choice

1/2 teaspoon ground turmeric

1/4 teaspoon ground cinnamon

1 tablespoon honey or maple syrup

1 tablespoon chopped almonds

Instructions:

In a saucepan, combine rolled oats, water or milk, turmeric, and cinnamon.

Bring to a boil, then reduce heat and simmer for 5-7 minutes, stirring occasionally, until oats are cooked and creamy.

Remove from heat and stir in honey or maple syrup.

Top with chopped almonds before serving.

Smoked Salmon and Avocado Bagel

Ingredients:

1 whole grain bagel, sliced and toasted

2 tablespoons cream cheese

2 slices smoked salmon

1/4 avocado, sliced

1 tablespoon capers (optional)

Instructions:

Spread cream cheese evenly on the toasted bagel halves.

Top each half with smoked salmon, avocado slices, and capers if using.

Serve immediately.

Greek Yogurt Parfait with Granola and Berries

Ingredients:

1/2 cup plain Greek yogurt

1/4 cup granola

1/4 cup mixed berries (such as strawberries, blueberries, and raspberries)

1 tablespoon honey or maple syrup

Instructions:

In a glass or bowl, layer Greek yogurt, granola, and mixed berries.

Drizzle with honey or maple syrup.

Serve immediately.

Egg and Vegetable Breakfast Wrap

Ingredients:

1 whole grain tortilla

2 eggs, scrambled

1/4 cup sautéed vegetables (such as spinach, bell peppers, onions, and mushrooms)

2 tablespoons shredded cheese (optional)

Salt and pepper to taste

Instructions:

Place scrambled eggs and sautéed vegetables in the center of the tortilla.

Sprinkle with shredded cheese if using.

Season with salt and pepper.

Roll up the tortilla to form a wrap.

Serve warm.

Chia Seed Pudding with Mango and Coconut

Ingredients:

2 tablespoons chia seeds

1/2 cup coconut milk

1/2 teaspoon vanilla extract

1/2 ripe mango, diced

1 tablespoon shredded coconut

Optional sweetener: honey, maple syrup, or stevia

Instructions:

In a bowl, combine chia seeds, coconut milk, and vanilla extract.

Stir well to combine, then let sit for 10-15 minutes to thicken.

Layer chia seed pudding with diced mango in serving glasses.

Top with shredded coconut and optional sweetener if desired.

Serve chilled.

Green Breakfast Bowl with Kale and Eggs

Ingredients:

1 cup cooked quinoa or brown rice

1 cup chopped kale, massaged with lemon juice

1 poached or fried egg

1/4 avocado, sliced

1 tablespoon pumpkin seeds

Salt and pepper to taste

Instructions:

In a bowl, layer cooked quinoa or brown rice with chopped kale.

Top with a poached or fried egg and sliced avocado.

Sprinkle with pumpkin seeds and season with salt and pepper.

Serve immediately.

Blueberry Almond Overnight Oats

Ingredients:

1/2 cup rolled oats

1/2 cup unsweetened almond milk

1/4 cup Greek yogurt

1/4 cup fresh or frozen blueberries

1 tablespoon almond butter

1 teaspoon honey or maple syrup

Instructions:

In a jar or container, combine rolled oats, almond milk, Greek yogurt, blueberries, almond butter, and honey or maple syrup.

Stir well to combine, then cover and refrigerate overnight.

In the morning, give the oats a good stir, then enjoy cold or warm.

These breakfast recipes are not only delicious but also packed with nutrients that can help support overall health and reduce the risk of cancer. Feel free to customize the recipes based on your preferences and dietary needs.

Lunch Recipes

Here are some lunch recipes tailored to the Starve cancer with food, featuring nutrient-rich ingredients and cancer-fighting properties:

Quinoa Salad with Chickpeas and Avocado

Ingredients:

1 cup cooked quinoa

1/2 cup cooked chickpeas

1/2 avocado, diced

1/4 cup cherry tomatoes, halved

1/4 cup cucumber, diced

2 tablespoons fresh parsley, chopped

1 tablespoon olive oil

1 tablespoon lemon juice

Salt and pepper to taste

Instructions:

In a large bowl, combine cooked quinoa, chickpeas, avocado, cherry tomatoes, cucumber, and parsley.

Drizzle with olive oil and lemon juice.

Season with salt and pepper, then toss gently to combine.

Serve chilled or at room temperature.

Salmon and Vegetable Stir-Fry

Ingredients:

1 tablespoon olive oil

1/2 pound salmon fillet, cut into chunks

2 cups mixed vegetables (such as bell peppers, broccoli, snap peas, and carrots)

2 cloves garlic, minced

1 tablespoon low-sodium soy sauce

1 teaspoon sesame oil

1/2 teaspoon grated ginger

Cooked brown rice or quinoa for serving

Instructions:

Heat olive oil in a large skillet or wok over medium-high heat.

Add salmon chunks and cook for 3-4 minutes until browned on all sides.

Add mixed vegetables and minced garlic to the skillet.

Stir-fry for 5-6 minutes until vegetables are tender-crisp.

In a small bowl, whisk together soy sauce, sesame oil, and grated ginger.

Pour the sauce over the salmon and vegetables, then toss to coat.

Serve the stir-fry over cooked brown rice or quinoa.

Mediterranean Chickpea Salad

Ingredients:

1 can (15 oz) chickpeas, drained and rinsed

1/2 cup cucumber, diced

1/2 cup cherry tomatoes, halved

1/4 cup red onion, diced

1/4 cup Kalamata olives, pitted and sliced

2 tablespoons feta cheese, crumbled

2 tablespoons fresh parsley, chopped

1 tablespoon olive oil

1 tablespoon lemon juice

Salt and pepper to taste

Instructions:

In a large bowl, combine chickpeas, cucumber, cherry tomatoes, red onion, olives, feta cheese, and parsley.

Drizzle with olive oil and lemon juice.

Season with salt and pepper, then toss gently to combine.

Serve chilled or at room temperature.

Grilled Chicken and Vegetable Skewers

Ingredients:

1 pound boneless, skinless chicken breast, cut into chunks

1 bell pepper, cut into chunks

1 zucchini, sliced

1 red onion, cut into chunks

1 tablespoon olive oil

1 tablespoon balsamic vinegar

1 teaspoon dried herbs (such as thyme, rosemary, or oregano)

Salt and pepper to taste

Instructions:

Preheat grill or grill pan to medium-high heat.

In a bowl, toss chicken chunks, bell pepper, zucchini, and red onion with olive oil, balsamic vinegar, dried herbs, salt, and pepper.

Thread chicken and vegetables onto skewers, alternating ingredients.

Grill skewers for 10-12 minutes, turning occasionally, until chicken is cooked through and vegetables are tender.

Serve hot with a side salad or whole grain bread.

Soba Noodle Salad with Edamame and Peanut Dressing

Ingredients:

6 oz soba noodles, cooked according to package instructions

1 cup shelled edamame, cooked

1/2 cup shredded carrots

1/4 cup sliced green onions

2 tablespoons chopped cilantro

2 tablespoons chopped peanuts

For the dressing:

2 tablespoons peanut butter

2 tablespoons soy sauce

1 tablespoon rice vinegar

1 tablespoon sesame oil

1 teaspoon honey or maple syrup

1 teaspoon grated ginger

1 clove garlic, minced

Instructions:

In a large bowl, combine cooked soba noodles, edamame, shredded carrots, green onions, and cilantro.

In a small bowl, whisk together peanut butter, soy sauce, rice vinegar, sesame oil, honey or maple syrup, grated ginger, and minced garlic to make the dressing.

Pour the dressing over the noodle salad and toss gently to coat.

Sprinkle chopped peanuts on top before serving.

Turkey and Avocado Wrap

Ingredients:

1 whole grain tortilla

3 oz sliced turkey breast

1/4 avocado, mashed

1/4 cup mixed greens

1 tablespoon hummus

1 teaspoon Dijon mustard

Instructions:

Spread mashed avocado evenly on the whole grain tortilla.

Layer sliced turkey breast, mixed greens, and hummus on top.

Drizzle with Dijon mustard.

Roll up the tortilla to form a wrap.

Serve immediately.

Roasted Vegetable Quinoa Bowl

Ingredients:

1 cup cooked quinoa

1 cup mixed roasted vegetables (such as sweet potatoes, Brussels sprouts, cauliflower, and broccoli)

1/4 cup crumbled feta cheese

2 tablespoons chopped walnuts

2 tablespoons balsamic glaze

Salt and pepper to taste

Instructions:

In a bowl, combine cooked quinoa and mix roasted vegetables.

Top with crumbled feta cheese and chopped walnuts.

Drizzle with balsamic glaze.

Season with salt and pepper, then toss gently to combine.

Serve warm or at room temperature.

Tuna Salad Stuffed Bell Peppers

Ingredients:

2 large bell peppers, halved and seeds removed

1 can (5 oz) tuna, drained

1/4 cup Greek yogurt

1/4 cup diced celery

2 tablespoons diced red onion

1 tablespoon lemon juice

1 teaspoon Dijon mustard

Salt and pepper to taste

Instructions:

Preheat oven to 375°F (190°C).

In a bowl, combine drained tuna, Greek yogurt, diced celery, diced red onion, lemon juice, Dijon mustard, salt, and pepper.

Spoon the tuna salad mixture into halved bell peppers.

Place stuffed bell peppers on a baking sheet lined with parchment paper.

Bake for 20-25 minutes until peppers are tender and filling is heated through.

Serve hot or chilled.

Spinach and Feta Stuffed Portobello Mushrooms

Ingredients:

4 large portobello mushrooms, stems removed

2 cups fresh spinach leaves

1/4 cup crumbled feta cheese

2 tablespoons chopped sun-dried tomatoes

2 cloves garlic, minced

1 tablespoon olive oil

Salt and pepper to taste

Instructions:

Preheat oven to 375°F (190°C).

In a skillet, heat olive oil over medium heat.

Add minced garlic and cook for 1-2 minutes until fragrant.

Add fresh spinach leaves to the skillet and cook until wilted.

Remove from heat and stir in crumbled feta cheese and chopped sun-dried tomatoes.

Season with salt and pepper to taste.

Stuff each portobello mushroom with the spinach mixture.

Place stuffed mushrooms on a baking sheet lined with parchment paper.

Bake for 15-20 minutes until mushrooms are tender.

Serve hot.

Black Bean and Quinoa Salad with Lime Dressing

Ingredients:

1 cup cooked quinoa

1 can (15 oz) black beans, drained and rinsed

1/2 cup diced red bell pepper

1/4 cup diced red onion

1/4 cup chopped cilantro

Juice of 2 limes

2 tablespoons olive oil

1 teaspoon honey or maple syrup

Salt and pepper to taste

Instructions:

In a large bowl, combine cooked quinoa, black beans, diced red bell pepper, diced red onion, and chopped cilantro.

In a small bowl, whisk together lime juice, olive oil, honey or maple syrup, salt, and pepper to make the dressing.

Pour the dressing over the quinoa salad and toss gently to coat.

Serve chilled or at room temperature.

These lunch recipes are not only delicious but also packed with nutrients that can help support overall health and reduce the risk of cancer. Feel free to customize the recipes based on your preferences and dietary needs.

Dinner Recipes

Here are some dinner recipes aligned with Anti-Cancer Diet:

Grilled Salmon with Quinoa and Steamed Broccoli

Ingredients:

2 salmon fillets

1 cup cooked quinoa

2 cups broccoli florets

Olive oil

Lemon slices

Salt and pepper

Instructions:

Preheat grill to medium-high heat.

Brush salmon fillets with olive oil and season with salt and pepper.

Grill salmon for 4-5 minutes per side, or until cooked through.

Meanwhile, steam broccoli until tender.

Serve grilled salmon with cooked quinoa, steamed broccoli, and lemon slices.

Vegetable Stir-Fry with Tofu

Ingredients:

1 block firm tofu, pressed and cubed

2 cups mixed vegetables (bell peppers, broccoli, snap peas, carrots)

2 cloves garlic, minced

2 tablespoons low-sodium soy sauce

1 tablespoon sesame oil

Cooked brown rice or quinoa

Sesame seeds for garnish

Instructions:

Heat sesame oil in a large skillet or wok over medium heat.

Add cubed tofu and cook until golden brown on all sides.

Add minced garlic and mixed vegetables to the skillet.

Stir-fry until vegetables are tender-crisp.

Stir in soy sauce and cook for an additional minute.

Serve vegetable stir-fry over cooked brown rice or quinoa, garnished with sesame seeds.

Lentil and Vegetable Soup

Ingredients:

1 cup dry lentils, rinsed

4 cups vegetable broth

2 cups diced tomatoes

2 cups mixed vegetables (carrots, celery, onion, kale)

2 cloves garlic, minced

1 teaspoon dried thyme

Salt and pepper to taste

Instructions:

In a large pot, combine lentils, vegetable broth, diced tomatoes, mixed vegetables, minced garlic, and dried thyme.

Bring to a boil, then reduce heat and simmer for 20-25 minutes, or until lentils are tender.

Season with salt and pepper to taste.

Serve hot, garnished with fresh herbs if desired.

Grilled Chicken Salad with Balsamic Vinaigrette

Ingredients:

2 boneless, skinless chicken breasts

Mixed salad greens

Cherry tomatoes, halved

Cucumber, sliced

Red onion, thinly sliced

Balsamic vinaigrette dressing

Instructions:

Preheat grill to medium-high heat.

Season chicken breasts with salt and pepper.

Grill chicken for 6-8 minutes per side, or until cooked through.

Let chicken rest for a few minutes, then slice.

Arrange mixed salad greens, cherry tomatoes, cucumber slices, and red onion on plates.

Top with sliced grilled chicken.

Drizzle with balsamic vinaigrette dressing.

Vegetable and Chickpea Curry

Ingredients:

1 tablespoon coconut oil

1 onion, diced

2 cloves garlic, minced

1 tablespoon grated ginger

2 tablespoons curry powder

1 can (15 oz) chickpeas, drained and rinsed

2 cups diced tomatoes

2 cups mixed vegetables (such as cauliflower, bell peppers, and spinach)

1 can (14 oz) coconut milk

Salt and pepper to taste

Cooked brown rice for serving

Instructions:

Heat coconut oil in a large pot over medium heat.

Add diced onion, minced garlic, and grated ginger to the pot.

Cook until onion is softened, about 5 minutes.

Stir in curry powder and cook for an additional minute.

Add chickpeas, diced tomatoes, mixed vegetables, and coconut milk to the pot.

Bring to a simmer and cook for 15-20 minutes, or until vegetables are tender.

Season with salt and pepper to taste.

Serve vegetable and chickpea curry over cooked brown rice.

Baked Cod with Lemon and Herbs

Ingredients:

4 cod fillets

2 tablespoons olive oil

2 tablespoons fresh lemon juice

2 cloves garlic, minced

1 teaspoon dried thyme

1 teaspoon dried rosemary

Salt and pepper to taste

Instructions:

Preheat oven to 400°F (200°C).

Place cod fillets in a baking dish.

In a small bowl, whisk together olive oil, lemon juice, minced garlic, dried thyme, dried rosemary, salt, and pepper.

Pour the lemon and herb mixture over the cod fillets.

Bake for 12-15 minutes, or until fish is cooked through and flakes easily with a fork.

Serve hot, garnished with fresh herbs if desired.

Vegetarian Stuffed Bell Peppers

Ingredients:

4 bell peppers, halved and seeds removed

1 cup cooked quinoa

1 can (15 oz) black beans, drained and rinsed

1 cup diced tomatoes

1 cup corn kernels

1/2 cup shredded cheese

1 teaspoon chili powder

1/2 teaspoon cumin

Salt and pepper to taste

Instructions:

Preheat oven to 375°F (190°C).

Place bell pepper halves in a baking dish.

In a large bowl, combine cooked quinoa, black beans, diced tomatoes, corn kernels, shredded cheese, chili powder, cumin, salt, and pepper.

Spoon the quinoa mixture into the bell pepper halves.

Cover the baking dish with foil and bake for 30-35 minutes, or until peppers are tender.

Serve hot, garnished with fresh herbs if desired.

Eggplant and Chickpea Curry

Ingredients:

1 eggplant, diced

1 can (15 oz) chickpeas, drained and rinsed

1 onion, diced

2 cloves garlic, minced

1 tablespoon grated ginger

1 tablespoon curry powder

1 can (14 oz) diced tomatoes

1 can (14 oz) coconut milk

2 tablespoons chopped cilantro

Cooked brown rice for serving

Salt and pepper to taste

Instructions:

Heat olive oil in a large pot over medium heat.

Add diced onion, minced garlic, and grated ginger to the pot.

Cook until onion is softened, about 5 minutes.

Stir in curry powder and cook for an additional minute.

Add diced eggplant, chickpeas, diced tomatoes, and coconut milk to the pot.

Bring to a simmer and cook for 20-25 minutes, or until eggplant is tender.

Season with salt and pepper to taste.

Serve eggplant and chickpea curry over cooked brown rice, garnished with chopped cilantro.

Spinach and Mushroom Frittata

Ingredients:

8 eggs

1 cup baby spinach leaves

1 cup sliced mushrooms

1/2 onion, diced

1/2 cup shredded cheese

1 tablespoon olive oil

Salt and pepper to taste

Instructions:

Preheat oven to 350°F (175°C).

Heat olive oil in a large oven-safe skillet over medium heat.

Add diced onion and sliced mushrooms to the skillet.

Cook until vegetables are softened, about 5 minutes.

Add baby spinach leaves to the skillet and cook until wilted.

In a bowl, whisk together eggs, shredded cheese, salt, and pepper.

Pour the egg mixture into the skillet over the cooked vegetables.

Cook for 3-4 minutes, or until the edges start to set.

Transfer the skillet to the preheated oven and bake for 15-20 minutes, or until the frittata is set in the center.

Serve hot or at room temperature.

Sesame Ginger Tofu Stir-Fry

Ingredients:

1 block of firm tofu, pressed and cubed

2 cups mixed vegetables (bell peppers, broccoli, snap peas, carrots)

2 cloves garlic, minced

2 tablespoons low-sodium soy sauce

1 tablespoon sesame oil

1 tablespoon grated ginger

1 tablespoon sesame seeds

Cooked brown rice or quinoa

Instructions:

Heat sesame oil in a large skillet or wok over medium heat.

Add cubed tofu and cook until golden brown on all sides.

Add minced garlic and mixed vegetables to the skillet.

Stir-fry until vegetables are tender-crisp.

In a small bowl, whisk together soy sauce and grated ginger.

Pour the sauce over the tofu and vegetables, then toss to coat.

Sprinkle sesame seeds on top before serving.

95 | STARVE CANCER WITH FOOD

Serve the stir-fry over cooked brown rice or quinoa.

These dinner recipes are not only delicious but also incorporate cancer-fighting ingredients to support overall health and well-being. Feel free to adjust the recipes according to your taste preferences and dietary needs. Enjoy your meals!

Snacks and Side Dishes Recipes

Here are some snacks and side dishes recipes suitable for the starving cancer with food:

Hummus and Vegetable Crudites

Ingredients:

1 cup chickpeas, drained and rinsed

2 tablespoons tahini

2 tablespoons lemon juice

1 clove garlic, minced

2 tablespoons olive oil

Salt and pepper to taste

Assorted vegetable for dipping (carrot sticks, cucumber slices, bell pepper strips)

Instructions:

In a food processor, combine chickpeas, tahini, lemon juice, minced garlic, olive oil, salt, and pepper.

Blend until smooth and creamy, adding a splash of water if needed to reach desired consistency.

Serve hummus with assorted vegetable crudites for dipping.

Edamame with Sea Salt

Ingredients:

1 cup edamame, cooked and shelled

Sea salt to taste

97 | STARVE CANCER WITH FOOD

Instructions:

Bring a pot of water to a boil and cook edamame according to package instructions.

Drain and rinse edamame under cold water.

Sprinkle with sea salt before serving as a nutritious snack.

Greek Yogurt with Berries and Almonds

Ingredients:

1/2 cup plain Greek yogurt

1/4 cup mixed berries (such as strawberries, blueberries, and raspberries)

1 tablespoon chopped almonds

Drizzle of honey or maple syrup (optional)

Instructions:

Spoon Greek yogurt into a bowl.

Top with mixed berries and chopped almonds.

Drizzle with honey or maple syrup if desired.

Roasted Chickpeas

Ingredients:

1 can (15 oz) chickpeas, drained and rinsed

1 tablespoon olive oil

1 teaspoon paprika

1/2 teaspoon cumin

1/2 teaspoon garlic powder

Salt to taste

Instructions:

Preheat oven to 400°F (200°C).

Pat chickpeas dry with a paper towel and remove any loose skins.

In a bowl, toss chickpeas with olive oil, paprika, cumin, garlic powder, and salt until evenly coated.

Spread chickpeas in a single layer on a baking sheet lined with parchment paper.

Roast for 25-30 minutes, shaking the pan halfway through, until chickpeas are crispy.

Let cool before serving as a crunchy snack.

Stuffed Bell Pepper Rings

Ingredients:

2 bell peppers, sliced into rings

1/2 cup hummus

1/4 cup diced cucumber

1/4 cup diced tomato

1 tablespoon chopped fresh parsley

Instructions:

Arrange bell pepper rings on a serving platter.

Fill each bell pepper ring with a spoonful of hummus.

100 | STARVE CANCER WITH FOOD

Top with diced cucumber, diced tomato, and chopped fresh parsley.

Serve as a colorful and flavorful side dish or snack.

Caprese Salad Skewers

Ingredients:

Cherry tomatoes

Fresh mozzarella balls

Fresh basil leaves

Balsamic glaze

Toothpicks

Instructions:

Thread a cherry tomato, a mozzarella ball, and a fresh basil leaf onto each toothpick.

Arrange the skewers on a serving platter.

Drizzle with balsamic glaze just before serving.

Cucumber and Tomato Salad

Ingredients:

2 cucumbers, diced

2 tomatoes, diced

1/4 red onion, thinly sliced

2 tablespoons chopped fresh parsley

1 tablespoon olive oil

1 tablespoon red wine vinegar

Salt and pepper to taste

Instructions:

In a large bowl, combine diced cucumbers, diced tomatoes, sliced red onion, and chopped fresh parsley.

Drizzle with olive oil and red wine vinegar.

Season with salt and pepper, then toss gently to combine.

Serve chilled as a refreshing side dish.

Kale Chips

Ingredients:

1 bunch kale, stems removed and torn into bite-sized pieces

1 tablespoon olive oil

Salt to taste

Instructions:

Preheat oven to 350°F (175°C).

In a large bowl, toss kale pieces with olive oil until evenly coated.

Spread kale in a single layer on a baking sheet lined with parchment paper.

Sprinkle with salt.

Bake for 10-15 minutes, or until kale is crispy but not burnt.

Let cool before serving as a crunchy snack.

Quinoa and Black Bean Salad

Ingredients:

1 cup cooked quinoa

1 can (15 oz) black beans, drained and rinsed

1/2 red bell pepper, diced

1/2 yellow bell pepper, diced

1/4 cup diced red onion

2 tablespoons chopped fresh cilantro

Juice of 1 lime

1 tablespoon olive oil

Salt and pepper to taste

Instructions:

In a large bowl, combine cooked quinoa, black beans, diced bell peppers, diced red onion, and chopped fresh cilantro.

Drizzle with lime juice and olive oil.

Season with salt and pepper, then toss gently to combine.

Serve chilled as a nutritious side dish or snack.

Fruit Salad with Mint-Lime Dressing

Ingredients:

Assorted fresh fruits (such as berries, melon, pineapple, and grapes), diced

Fresh mint leaves, chopped

Juice of 1 lime

1 tablespoon honey or maple syrup (optional)

Instructions:

In a large bowl, combine diced fresh fruits and chopped fresh mint leaves.

Drizzle with lime juice and honey or maple syrup if desired.

Toss gently to combine.

Serve chilled as a refreshing snack or side dish.

These snacks and side dishes are not only delicious but also packed with nutrients to support overall health and well-being. Enjoy them as part of your Anti-Cancer Diet!

Herb Recipes

Here are some herb-infused recipes suitable for the Anti-Cancer Diet:

Herb-Crusted Baked Salmon

Ingredients:

4 salmon fillets

2 tablespoons chopped fresh parsley

1 tablespoon chopped fresh dill

1 tablespoon chopped fresh chives

1 tablespoon lemon zest

2 cloves garlic, minced

2 tablespoons olive oil

Salt and pepper to taste

Instructions:

Preheat oven to 375°F (190°C) and line a baking sheet with parchment paper.

In a small bowl, combine chopped parsley, dill, chives, lemon zest, minced garlic, olive oil, salt, and pepper.

Pat the salmon fillets dry with a paper towel and place them on the prepared baking sheet.

Spread the herb mixture evenly over the top of each salmon fillet.

Bake for 12-15 minutes, or until salmon is cooked through and flakes easily with a fork.

Serve hot with your favorite side dishes.

Garlic and Herb Roasted Vegetables

Ingredients:

Assorted vegetables (such as carrots, potatoes, bell peppers, and zucchini), cut into chunks

3 cloves garlic, minced

2 tablespoons chopped fresh rosemary

2 tablespoons chopped fresh thyme

2 tablespoons olive oil

Salt and pepper to taste

Instructions:

Preheat oven to 400°F (200°C) and line a baking sheet with parchment paper.

In a large bowl, toss the assorted vegetables with minced garlic, chopped rosemary, chopped thyme, olive oil, salt, and pepper until evenly coated.

Spread the seasoned vegetables in a single layer on the prepared baking sheet.

Roast for 25-30 minutes, or until vegetables are tender and caramelized.

Serve hot as a flavorful side dish.

Herb-Marinated Grilled Chicken

Ingredients:

4 boneless, skinless chicken breasts

1/4 cup chopped fresh basil

1/4 cup chopped fresh parsley

2 tablespoons chopped fresh oregano

2 cloves garlic, minced

1/4 cup olive oil

Juice of 1 lemon

Salt and pepper to taste

Instructions:

109 | STARVE CANCER WITH FOOD

In a small bowl, whisk together chopped basil, parsley, oregano, minced garlic, olive oil, lemon juice, salt, and pepper to make the marinade.

Place chicken breasts in a resealable plastic bag and pour the marinade over them.

Seal the bag and massage the marinade into the chicken breasts.

Refrigerate for at least 30 minutes, or up to 4 hours.

Preheat grill to medium-high heat and lightly oil the grate.

Remove chicken breasts from the marinade and discard any excess marinade.

Grill chicken for 6-8 minutes per side, or until cooked through and no longer pink in the center.

Serve hot with your favorite grilled vegetables.

Lemon-Herb Quinoa Salad

Ingredients:

1 cup quinoa, rinsed

2 cups water or vegetable broth

1/4 cup chopped fresh parsley

2 tablespoons chopped fresh mint

2 tablespoons chopped fresh dill

1/4 cup olive oil

Juice of 2 lemons

Salt and pepper to taste

Optional add-ins: diced cucumber, cherry tomatoes, feta cheese

Instructions:

In a medium saucepan, combine quinoa and water or vegetable broth.

Bring to a boil, then reduce heat to low, cover, and simmer for 15-20 minutes, or until quinoa is cooked and liquid is absorbed.

Fluff quinoa with a fork and transfer it to a large bowl to cool slightly.

In a small bowl, whisk together chopped parsley, mint, dill, olive oil, lemon juice, salt, and pepper to make the dressing.

Pour the dressing over the cooked quinoa and toss to combine.

Stir in any optional add-ins, if desired.

Serve the quinoa salad warm or chilled.

Herb-Roasted Cherry Tomatoes

Ingredients:

2 cups cherry tomatoes, halved

2 tablespoons chopped fresh basil

2 tablespoons chopped fresh thyme

2 tablespoons olive oil

Salt and pepper to taste

Instructions:

Preheat oven to 400°F (200°C) and line a baking sheet with parchment paper.

In a bowl, toss cherry tomato halves with chopped basil, thyme, olive oil, salt, and pepper until evenly coated.

Spread the seasoned cherry tomatoes in a single layer on the prepared baking sheet.

Roast for 15-20 minutes, or until tomatoes are blistered and caramelized.

Serve hot as a flavorful side dish or topping for salads and pasta.

Herb-Infused Olive Oil

Ingredients:

1 cup extra virgin olive oil

4 cloves garlic, peeled and smashed

2 sprigs fresh rosemary

4 sprigs fresh thyme

2 dried red chili peppers (optional)

Instructions:

In a small saucepan, combine olive oil, smashed garlic cloves, rosemary sprigs, thyme sprigs, and dried red chili peppers (if using).

Heat the mixture over low heat until garlic starts to sizzle, then remove from heat and let cool completely.

Transfer the infused olive oil to a clean glass bottle or jar, using a fine-mesh strainer to remove solids.

Seal the bottle or jar tightly and store in a cool, dark place for up to 2 weeks.

Use the herb-infused olive oil for drizzling over salads, dipping bread, or marinating vegetables and meats.

Herb-Roasted Potatoes

Ingredients:

1 pound baby potatoes, halved or quartered

2 tablespoons chopped fresh rosemary

2 tablespoons chopped fresh thyme

2 tablespoons chopped fresh parsley

2 cloves garlic, minced

2 tablespoons olive oil

Salt and pepper to taste

Instructions:

Preheat oven to 400°F (200°C) and line a baking sheet with parchment paper.

In a large bowl, toss halved baby potatoes with chopped rosemary, thyme, parsley, minced garlic, olive oil, salt, and pepper until evenly coated.

Spread the seasoned potatoes in a single layer on the prepared baking sheet.

Roast for 25-30 minutes, or until potatoes are golden brown and crispy on the outside and tender on the inside.

Serve hot as a delicious side dish.

Herb-Marinated Grilled Vegetables

Ingredients:

Assorted vegetables (such as zucchini, eggplant, bell peppers, and mushrooms), sliced

1/4 cup chopped fresh basil

1/4 cup chopped fresh parsley

2 tablespoons chopped fresh oregano

2 cloves garlic, minced

1/4 cup olive oil

Juice of 1 lemon

Salt and pepper to taste

Instructions:

In a large bowl, combine sliced vegetables with chopped basil, parsley, oregano, minced garlic, olive oil, lemon juice, salt, and pepper.

Toss until the vegetables are evenly coated with the herb marinade.

Let the vegetables marinate for at least 30 minutes, or up to 2 hours, in the refrigerator.

Preheat grill to medium-high heat and lightly oil the grate.

Remove vegetables from the marinade and thread them onto skewers.

Grill the skewers for 8-10 minutes, turning occasionally, until vegetables are tender and lightly charred.

Serve hot as a flavorful side dish or as a vegetarian main course.

Herb and Garlic Cauliflower Mash

Ingredients:

1 head cauliflower, cut into florets

2 cloves garlic, minced

2 tablespoons chopped fresh parsley

2 tablespoons chopped fresh chives

2 tablespoons olive oil

Salt and pepper to taste

Instructions:

Bring a large pot of salted water to a boil.

Add cauliflower florets to the boiling water and cook for 8-10 minutes, or until tender.

Drain cauliflower and transfer it to a food processor.

Add minced garlic, chopped parsley, chopped chives, olive oil, salt, and pepper to the food processor.

Pulse until cauliflower is smooth and creamy, scraping down the sides of the bowl as needed.

Adjust seasoning to taste.

Serve hot as a nutritious side dish.

Herb and Lemon Rice Pilaf

Ingredients:

1 cup basmati rice

2 cups vegetable broth

2 tablespoons chopped fresh dill

2 tablespoons chopped fresh parsley

1 tablespoon chopped fresh chives

Zest of 1 lemon

2 tablespoons olive oil

Salt and pepper to taste

Instructions:

Rinse basmati rice under cold water until the water runs clear.

In a saucepan, combine rinsed rice, vegetable broth, chopped dill, chopped parsley, chopped chives, lemon zest, olive oil, salt, and pepper.

Bring to a boil, then reduce heat to low, cover, and simmer for 15-20 minutes, or until rice is cooked and liquid is absorbed.

Fluff rice with a fork and adjust seasoning to taste.

Serve hot as a fragrant and flavorful side dish.

These herb-infused recipes add a burst of flavor and freshness to your meals while providing essential nutrients to support your overall health and well-being. Enjoy incorporating them into your Anti-Cancer Diet!

121 | STARVE CANCER WITH FOOD

Chapter Five

One-Week Meal Plan for Beginners

Here's a sample one-week meal plan suitable for beginners following the starve cancer with food. Each day includes three main meals and two snacks, incorporating a variety of nutrient-rich foods and cancer-fighting ingredients:

Day 1

Breakfast: Herb and Garlic Cauliflower Mash

Snack: Greek Yogurt with Berries and Almonds

Lunch: Herb-Marinated Grilled Chicken with Lemon-Herb Quinoa Salad

Snack: Hummus and Vegetable Crudites

Dinner: Herb-Crusted Baked Salmon with Roasted Garlic and Herb Potatoes

Day 2

Breakfast: Lemon-Herb Rice Pilaf

Snack: Edamame with Sea Salt

Lunch: Herb and Lemon Rice Pilaf with Herb-Roasted Cherry Tomatoes

Snack: Caprese Salad Skewers

Dinner: Garlic and Herb Roasted Vegetables with Sesame Ginger Tofu Stir-Fry

Day 3

Breakfast: Herb and Garlic Cauliflower Mash

Snack: Fruit Salad with Mint-Lime Dressing

Lunch: Herb-Marinated Grilled Vegetables with Quinoa and Black Bean Salad

Snack: Herb-Infused Olive Oil with Whole Grain Bread

Dinner: Herb-Crusted Baked Salmon with Spinach and Mushroom Frittata

Day 4

Breakfast: Lemon-Herb Rice Pilaf

Snack: Roasted Chickpeas

Lunch: Greek Yogurt with Berries and Almonds

Snack: Stuffed Bell Pepper Rings

Dinner: Herb-Marinated Grilled Chicken with Herb and Lemon Rice Pilaf

Day 5

Breakfast: Herb and Garlic Cauliflower Mash

Snack: Greek Yogurt with Berries and Almonds

Lunch: Herb-Roasted Potatoes with Lentil and Herb Soup

Snack: Edamame with Sea Salt

Dinner: Garlic and Herb Roasted Vegetables with Herb-Crusted Baked Salmon

Day 6

Breakfast: Lemon-Herb Rice Pilaf

Snack: Fruit Salad with Mint-Lime Dressing

Lunch: Herb-Crusted Baked Salmon with Spinach and Mushroom Frittata

Snack: Caprese Salad Skewers

Dinner: Herb-Marinated Grilled Vegetables with Quinoa and Black Bean Salad

Day 7

Breakfast: Herb and Garlic Cauliflower Mash

Snack: Roasted Chickpeas

125 | STARVE CANCER WITH FOOD

Lunch: Greek Yogurt with Berries and Almonds

Snack: Hummus and Vegetable Crudites

Dinner: Garlic and Herb Roasted Vegetables with Sesame Ginger Tofu Stir-Fry

This one-week meal plan provides a variety of delicious and nutritious meals while incorporating cancer-fighting herbs and ingredients. Feel free to adjust portion sizes and ingredients to suit your preferences and dietary needs.

Tips for Dining Out and Socializing

Navigating dining out and socializing while following an anti-cancer diet can be challenging, but with some planning and awareness, it's entirely feasible.

Here are some tips to help you make healthier choices and enjoy social occasions without compromising your dietary goals:

1. Research Restaurants in Advance:

Before heading out, look up the restaurant's menu online to see if they offer healthy options that align with your dietary preferences. Many restaurants now provide nutritional information alongside their menus, which can help you make informed choices.

2. Choose Restaurants Wisely:

Opt for restaurants that prioritize fresh, whole ingredients and offer customizable dishes. Avoid fast food chains and opt for local eateries or farm-to-table restaurants that focus on quality ingredients.

3. Focus on Vegetables and Lean Proteins:

When ordering, prioritize dishes that are rich in vegetables and lean proteins. Look for grilled, steamed, or roasted options rather than fried or heavily processed dishes.

4. Watch Portion Sizes:

Pay attention to portion sizes, as restaurant servings tend to be larger than what you might eat at home. Consider sharing an entree with a friend or asking for a half portion if available.

5. Be Mindful of Cooking Methods:

Choose dishes that are prepared using healthier cooking methods such as grilling, steaming, or baking, and avoid dishes that are deep-fried or heavily sautéed in oil.

6. Customize Your Order:

Don't hesitate to customize your order to suit your dietary needs. Ask for dressings and sauces on the side, request substitutions for healthier options, and inquire about ingredient substitutions or omissions.

7. Practice Portion Control:

Be mindful of portion sizes and avoid overeating. Consider ordering an appetizer or side dish instead of a full entree, or ask for a to-go box at the beginning of the meal and portion out half of your meal to take home.

8. Stay Hydrated:

Drink plenty of water throughout the meal to stay hydrated and help control hunger. Avoid sugary beverages and opt for water, herbal tea, or sparkling water with lemon instead.

9. Practice Mindful Eating:

Take your time to savor each bite, chew slowly, and pay attention to hunger cues. Mindful eating can help prevent overeating and promote better digestion.

10. Enjoy the Social Aspect:

Remember that dining out is not just about the food but also about enjoying the company of others. Focus on the conversation and the experience rather than solely on the food.

11. Plan Ahead for Social Gatherings:

If you're attending a social gathering or event, offer to bring a dish that aligns with your dietary preferences. This ensures that you'll have at least one healthy option available.

12. Be Flexible and Forgiving:

While it's important to stick to your dietary goals as much as possible, it's also essential to be flexible and forgiving with yourself. If you indulge in an occasional treat or stray from your plan, don't dwell on it. Instead, focus on making healthier choices moving forward.

By following these tips and strategies, you can navigate dining out and socializing while staying true to your anti-cancer dietary goals. Remember to prioritize whole, nutrient-rich foods, stay mindful of portion sizes, and enjoy

the experience of sharing meals with friends
and loved ones.

Conclusion

In conclusion, the Starve cancer with food Cookbook serves as a comprehensive guide to adopting a dietary approach that supports overall health and well-being while also reducing the risk of cancer. Throughout this cookbook, we've explored the role of nutrition in cancer prevention and treatment, emphasizing the importance of whole foods, nutrient-rich ingredients, and cancer-fighting nutrients.

By incorporating a variety of fruits, vegetables, whole grains, lean proteins, and healthy fats into your meals, you can nourish your body with the essential nutrients it needs to thrive and support your immune system's ability to fight off cancer cells.

Additionally, by avoiding processed foods, excessive sugar, unhealthy fats, and other harmful substances, you can reduce inflammation in the body and create an environment that is less conducive to cancer growth and development.

The recipes included in this cookbook are designed to be delicious, satisfying, and easy to prepare, making it simple to incorporate anti-cancer foods into your daily diet. From breakfasts and snacks to main meals and desserts, each recipe is thoughtfully crafted to provide a balance of flavors and nutrients that support optimal health.

Furthermore, this cookbook provides valuable tips for dining out, socializing, meal planning, and meal prep, empowering you to make healthier choices in any situation and stay on track with your dietary goals.

Ultimately, the Starving Cancer With Food Cookbook is not just a collection of recipe but a comprehensive resource for anyone looking to take control of their health and reduce their risk of cancer through the power of nutrition.

By embracing the principles outlined in this cookbook and making mindful choices about the foods you eat, you can nourish your body, support your immune system, and take proactive steps towards a healthier, cancer-free future.